Reviews

"Magic Forest Hugging Tree is a unique, charming, refreshing, and inspiring book. Both children and adults will benefit from Laura Hoffman's useful techniques."

Ann Webster, PhD
Benson Henry Institute for Mind Body Medicine
Harvard Medical School
USA

~

"This is a magical book full of magical word pictures and images to help the young people in your personal and/or professional life take control...it helps them paint vibrantly colorful pictures in their minds...I will be using these scripts with the young-at-heart of all ages in my life."

Dr. Naftali Halberstadt
Senior CBT therapist
Academic Director, Training Center for Mind-Body Skills
Israel

Magic Forest Hugging Tree is a wonderful book to read to children by itself or with Laura Hoffman's recordings, which are available on Amazon and iTunes under the name, "Laura Hoffman: Children's Guided Imagery."

Laura has produced the following:

CDs available for download

> Children's Guided Imagery (© 2010 Laura Hoffman)
> Guided Imagery and Meditation (© 2010 Laura Hoffman)

Books

> Magic Forest Hugging Tree (© 2012 Laura Hoffman)

Additional copies of this book are available for purchase on Amazon and in select bookstores.

To contact Laura, visit www.hoffmancounseling.com.

Magic Forest Hugging Tree

Children's Guided Imagery

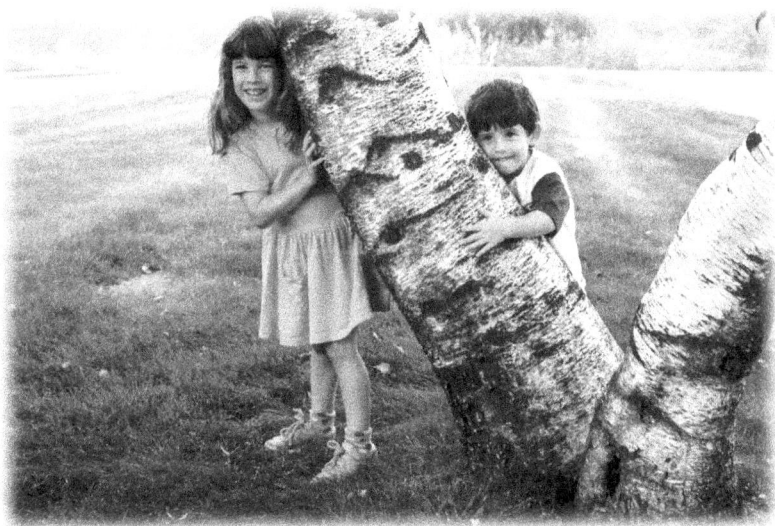

By Laura Hoffman

ISBN-13: 978-0615735009
ISBN-10: 0615735002

For Becky and Josh

My Heart Hugs and Inspiration

Acknowledgments

I would like to thank my family for offering the love and support I needed to complete this special book.

Thank you to my wonderful grown children, Josh and Becky, who always provide unconditional loving support and inspiration. Your editing and technical help has been instrumental in the creation of this book.

Thank you to my grandmother Helene who was my first holistic health teacher, and to my parents, Bob and Evie, who raised me to value health and healing of the mind-body-heart-spirit.

Thank you to all the children of the world whom I endeavor to help, one child at a time.

Contents

Script Summaries

Peace Tree

Make a special visit to meet the magical Peace Tree and leave all your troubles in the Worry Basket.

Magic Forest Hugging Tree

Come on a wonderful journey in the Magic Forest to meet the rabbit family and try out a cozy couch on your very own Hugging Tree.

Garden River

Visit the soothing Garden River where you will find a beautiful tree with special leaves to hold all your worries.

Heart Loving Rosebud

Feel the power of your loving heart! Imagine a beautiful rosebud bloom and share heart hugs with someone that you love.

Special Place

Imagine your very own Special Place where you feel safe and loved, and that you may visit anytime you choose.

Magic Rainbow

Join the happy little bird in playing "sliding down the bow" on the Magic Rainbow.

Be A Bird

Imagine you are a courageous little bird! Come take your first amazing flight.

Magic Mountain

Meet the magical Peace Tree on your journey as you climb to the top of the strong and powerful Magic Mountain.

Magic Star Ride

Come on a fun journey in the Magic Forest with the little bird, meet the magical Peace Tree, discover treasure and hop onto your very own Magic Star for a Magic Star ride.

Butterfly Garden

Make a magical visit to the Butterfly Garden and make new wonderful butterfly friends. What color butterfly are you?

Magic Garden

Welcome to the Magic Garden where you may plant your own vegetable garden. What is in your Magic Garden?

Energy Ball

Imagine an Energy Ball with tiny hearts, happy suns, glowing white light, a soft cloud or whatever YOU want.

Energy Shield

Imagine your very own Energy Shield. Create a safe space to help you feel powerful and protected. Learn to call up your Energy Shield whenever you need it.

One Minute Journey Summaries

Magic Fluffy Clouds

Imagine a fluffy cloud carrying away aches and pains.

Ball of Soothing Ice Water/Snow

Cool and soothe away aches and pains.

Rosebud

Feel beautiful, loving heart energy.

Heart Hug

Give yourself a loving heart hug.

Glowing Ball of Magical Light

Feel healing energy wash through your entire body.

Special Place

Create your own Special Place.

Energy Shields

Imagine three of your very own Energy Shields.

Introduction

Guided imagery has been shown to help children relieve pain, reduce stress and anxiety, find comfort, and promote healing. With guided imagery use, children may need less medication and experience fewer complications after surgery.

I wrote Magic Forest Hugging Tree out of a desire to reduce children's anxiety and lessen their pain by bringing them to safe, joyful and comforting places in their imaginations. These scripts offer the gift of unconditional love. They serve as a tool to help children develop strong minds and attain the personal power to feel calm within.

Children are born with a special gift of openness and the ability to tap into their innate capacity for healing. They amaze me with their ability to quickly enter relaxed and peaceful states while listening to my guided imagery scripts. I believe it is imperative to teach children, who may be anxious or in discomfort, skills to achieve independence and self-confidence by bringing peace and healing into their daily lives.

Over the decades, I have witnessed remarkable success for children using my guided imagery scripts and recordings, which I invite you to read, reread, memorize, and ultimately improvise upon. When reading to a child, speak in a calm and soothing voice that matches the rhythm of the script's words, and pause often to allow the child to fully experience the visualizations. These scripts are uniquely written to bring the child to a state of relaxation and peace. Encourage him or her to relax and thoroughly enjoy the experience.

Parents, caregivers, psychologists, medical staff, and educators are encouraged to read these guided imagery scripts to children before, during, and after surgery, as well as at home in daily life to create feelings of confidence, safety, comfort and love.

Magic Forest Hugging Tree is a special collection of my scripts that I now share with you and your children to offer many hours of relief, relaxation, healing, and joy. Use this book by itself or with my Children's Guided Imagery recordings.

I wish for you and your children a life of love, joy and beautiful imagining.

Note to Doctors, Nurses, Hospital Caregivers, Psychologists and Educators

I invite you to read these guided imagery scripts to child patients throughout their hospital stays. These scripts offer in-the-moment opportunities to create safe place imageries, helping children find immediate comfort in the face of fear, pain and difficult separations from loved ones.

For chronic pain situations, the full scripts may offer relief, healing and joy.

For acute situations, either reading the "One Minute Journeys" or reciting short phrases drawn from the full scripts may help a child cope with pain and lessen fear.

Please feel free to improvise upon the scripts in this book. Use your intuition and listen with an open mind to each child to decide which imagery will most benefit him or her. If a child loves a pet, person, toy, or color, encourage that child to include it during imagery.

Note to Parents

This is a book of comforting guided imagery scripts to read out loud to your child. If your child has trouble sleeping, feels anxious or fearful, experiences nervousness before taking medical tests or school exams, feels lonely or homesick, needs self confidence, experiences aches and pains, or simply needs a loving word, reading from this book may offer him or her comfort, unconditional love and a safe place.

I invite you to use the scripts in this book as a jump off point. Like the safe, cozy nest in the Be a Bird script from which the bird took its first flight, this book may help children gain confidence that allows their imaginations to grow, and develop strong minds for support throughout their lives.

I encourage you to move slowly through this book, inviting your child to participate and to add descriptions and responses as you read along while embracing the words and experience of each imagery. The clearer they see and feel the imagery, the more beneficial the overall experience will be. You may find emotional comfort from reading these scripts to your child at home or in the hospital by reducing fear and anxiety for your child and yourself. Your loving tone of voice will soothe you both.

A Special Note For Children

Welcome to the Magic Forest Hugging Tree book! I invite you to take a magical journey into a quiet and safe place in your imagination where you have the power to feel peaceful and joyful.

Not only will you imagine wonderful places and pictures in your mind, but you will also journey to fun places, such as the Hugging Tree and Peace Tree, where you feel safe, happy and loved. You are the boss of your own mind.

This magical book is a special gift for a grownup to read to you when you want to feel more relaxed and joyful.

When you relax and imagine, you are teaching yourself how to feel peaceful, strong and happy. These skills will benefit you throughout your life.

Enjoy this magical book, and welcome to Magic Forest Hugging Tree!

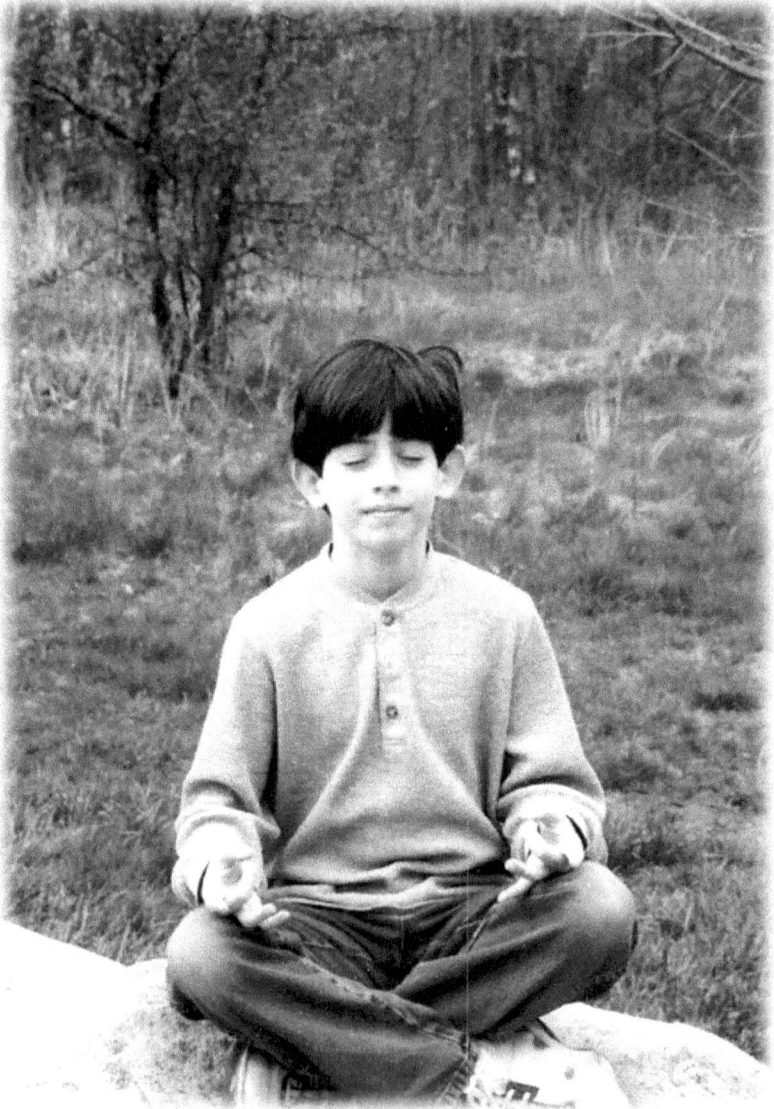

Scripts

Peace Tree

I invite you to come on a special journey to visit the Peace Tree.

Sometimes we have worries that make us feel a little anxious.

That's okay.

Did you know that you are able to make yourself feel better? You can let go of worries and instead imagine happy thoughts that make you peaceful! You can do this by imagining a visit to the Peace Tree.

Let's begin now by sitting in a comfortable space. This may be on a comfy chair or even outside somewhere in nature. To enjoy imagining, it is good to feel relaxed and quiet.

One way to quiet yourself is to close your eyes, place your hands on your belly and take a soft breath deep into your belly. Breathe in softly, then as you breathe out you can say a word to yourself like "peace" or "love." Your breath is your friend that helps you relax. Take three soft breaths into your belly now, and each time you breathe out say your word to yourself. This will help you quiet your mind.

Begin to relax the muscles of your body. Take a soft breath in and out and feel all the muscles of your body, from your head all the way to your toes, become soft and relaxed...just like pudding.

Imagine you are sitting on a grassy patch of earth next to a little river. This grassy patch of earth is very soft and cozy to sit on. Maybe you have a very soft blanket of your favorite color that is spread out on the grass. What color is your blanket? You see a little patch of flowers that smell wonderful. What color are the flowers?

Look! There is a big, beautiful tree right next to you. It is the Peace Tree and she is here for you to give her all your worries! Imagine that you give the Peace Tree a big hug.

There is a branch on the Peace Tree that is low enough for you to see a nest of birds that are singing and chirping because they are happy that you have arrived. What color are the birds?

You look up the tree trunk and into another low branch and see a special basket with your name on it. This is your very own Worry Basket. You climb easily up the Peace Tree trunk now and lean across the branch to get this basket. What color is your basket? Is it made of branches, wood or cloth? Is it big or small? The basket has a handle on it so it is easy for you to hold and carry with you as you climb back down to sit on your blanket in the grass.

There is a top on the basket and a little latch that you can open to see what is inside. Lift off the top of the basket and open it up now. Your Worry Basket is here for you to fill up with all your worries and any feelings that are troubling you.

Think about one thing that may be bothering you. Perhaps it is something that you are afraid of or worrying about. What is this one thing?

Whatever it is, you can tell this worry to go into the basket. You don't need to worry about it anymore. You can simply place it in the basket and close the top! Once this worry is in the basket, it will stay there until you give it permission to come out!

Think of another thing that you are worrying about. Again, you can place this worry in the basket right now and close the top!

Again, this worry will stay inside the basket until you give it permission to come out!

If there are any other worries, fears or troubles that you want to place in the basket, do it now. You have the power to put in as many worries as you want to.

After you finish this, close the top tightly and pat it softly. The Worry Basket is closed with all the worries and they can't come back out. The basket will always be big enough to hold them all.

Imagine that you carry your basket and climb back up the Peace Tree trunk to the branch where you found your basket. There is a place on the branch into which you put your basket. It fits perfectly.

This strong and powerful Peace Tree will now hold onto your basket of worries and troubles so you can be free to feel happy.

You climb back down, off the branch and down the tree trunk, and go back to your soft blanket on the grass.

All your worries and concerns are now gone and you feel free and happy. You are really proud of yourself!

You sit quietly on your spot next to the tree and see the little patch of flowers. They are facing towards the sun and are warm and beautiful. You look back up the Peace Tree at the branch with the birds. They are singing and chirping. They are proud of you and happy that you are here. You look at the little river of water next to the grass where you sit and notice colorful tiny fish swimming happily in the water.

You raise your arms and hands up to the sun and breathe a deep breath into your belly.

You have the power to make yourself feel better at any time.

Just imagine yourself visiting your Peace Tree and placing all your worries in your Worry Basket. You have the power to feel good.

Good for you!

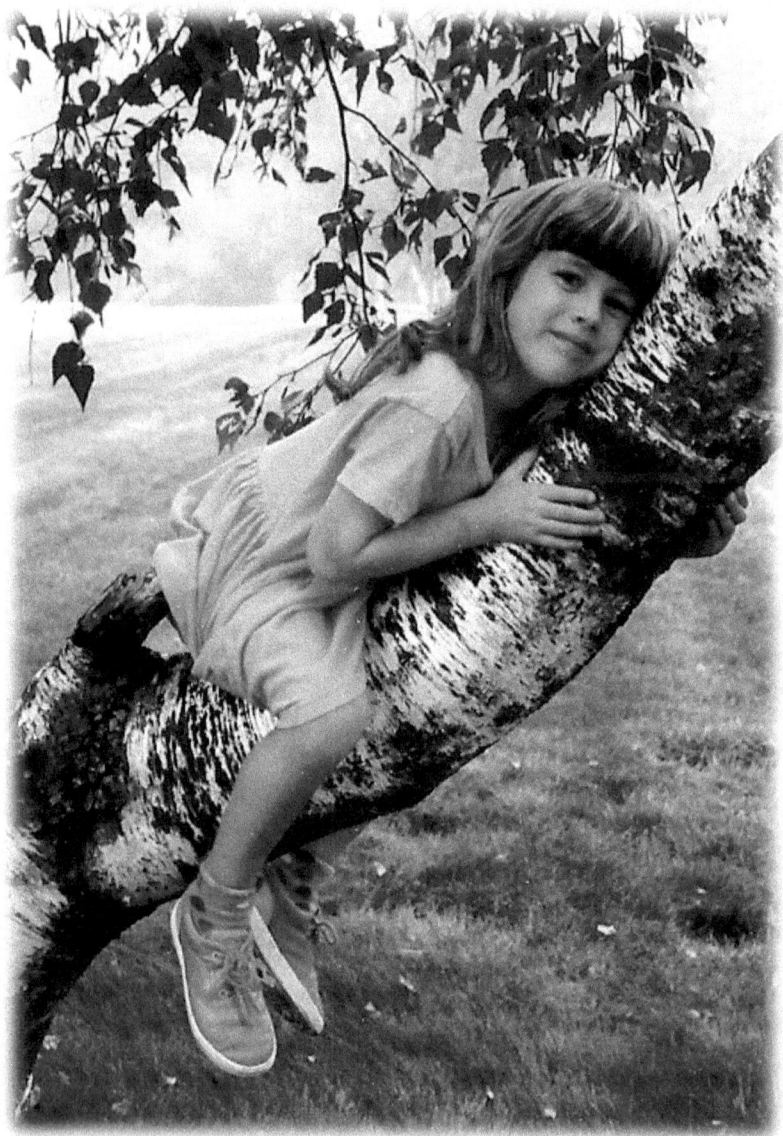

Magic Forest Hugging Tree

Imagine you are walking along a beautiful path in a Magic Forest. The earth feels soft under your feet as you walk. Perhaps you are wearing sandals or sneakers, or maybe you are barefoot.

You feel very happy as you walk along and wiggle and swing your arms all around.

There are bushes along the side of your path with little flowers on them. You stop next to one of the bushes to have a better look. You lean down to smell the flowers and are happily surprised to see a beautiful butterfly smiling up at you!

You say, "Good morning!" to the butterfly and watch her fly happily off to the next bush.

What color are the flowers on your bush? You gently touch the petals of one of the flowers. Do they feel soft or warm from the sunshine on them? Perhaps you can feel little dewdrops of water that are still on the petals from the early morning dew.

You take a deep breath, loving the aroma of the flowers, and continue to walk happily along your path.

You can see friendly trees of all sizes along your path and you wave to the trees as you go by. There is a gentle breeze in the forest and the branches and leaves of the trees look like they are waving back to you!

There is a special tree that you see right up ahead of you.

This is your very own Hugging Tree and it is so happy that you have arrived!

Your Hugging Tree is just the right size for you to give it a hug. Walk up to the tree now and spread your arms open wide. Take a deep breath into your belly, and as you breathe out give your tree a big hug.

What color or colors is your Hugging Tree? Notice how the bark on the trunk of the tree feels as you give it a hug. Perhaps it feels smooth and silky, or crinkly and hard. Does it feel warm from the sun shining on it? Can you put your arms all around the tree and touch your fingers together?

As you hug your special tree you can feel comforting energy. The tree is growing tall, strong and healthy just like you! Hug your tree as long as you like now.

You see in the bottom of the tree trunk a little opening. Curious, you bend down onto your knees and have a look inside the hole. It is easy for you to see inside because the rays of the sun are shining brightly onto the tree.

Look! There is a rabbit family inside the opening. You say, "Good morning." They are busy eating a breakfast of carrots and lettuce. They have little leaves the shape of cups from which they are sipping water. What colors are your rabbits?

One of the baby rabbits hops over to you and you reach your hand out to touch her soft fur. The rabbit touches your hand with her face. It tickles and makes you smile.

You are feeling so happy and satisfied right now.

The little rabbit hops back into the opening of the tree to continue eating breakfast with her family.

You look more closely at your Hugging Tree and notice a big tree root at the base of the tree that is just the right size for you to sit on. It is like a little couch that is here just for you. You settle down into the spot and lean against the tree.

You are feeling very relaxed and safe now as you sit in this special spot in your Hugging Tree.

As you curl up in this cozy spot, you can feel the leaves from some of the branches tickling your arms, just like a big hug! You are happy and satisfied and feel very loved right now. You can stay as long as you like, cuddled with your Hugging Tree.

If you like, you can imagine climbing around the tree and even up to one of the branches to explore. You find many spots in your Hugging Tree that are like little cozy couches for you to cuddle inside. Perhaps there are even blankets of leaves waiting here for you to sit on so that it is soft and cozy.

You try out many little cozy spots on your Hugging Tree and feel lots of hugs from the tree.

It is time now for you to leave your tree. You climb down the tree and peak into the little opening and say, "Goodbye," to the rabbits. They finished their breakfast and are curling up to have a nap.

You thank your Hugging Tree for being here for you and say, "Goodbye," to your special tree for now.

You know you can return to your special Hugging Tree anytime you want a hug.

You feel very loved, safe and "hugged" now as you walk back down the path in the Magic Forest.

You walk past the bush with the beautiful butterfly and stop to smell the lovely flowers again. You smile at the butterfly and say, "Goodbye," to this special Magic Forest.

You can return anytime you like in your imagination.

You are feeling loved and happy.

Take three breaths in and out of your belly now and feel proud of yourself!

Special Place

This is a time now for you to have a deep rest in your mind and body – a special time for you to feel safe and loved.

Begin to take some gentle breaths deep into your belly and as you breathe out, you can let go of all tension, allowing your muscles to feel soft and warm.

Breathe into the top of your head and feel the top of your head becoming soft and relaxed. Breathe into your forehead now as though a gentle breeze is soothing all the worry knots away.

Breathe into your eyes, relaxing all the muscles around your eyes. Breathe softness and warmth into your cheeks, your mouth and your neck. Feel all the tension wash out of your body so it feels relaxed and warm.

Breathe into your shoulders and feel all the tension rolling off your shoulders. Breathe down your arms, and breathe warmth into your hands and fingers.

Breathe into your chest and feel your chest becoming soft and comfortable. Breathe into your heart and feel your heart expanding while love and warmth come out.

Breathe into your belly; breathe warmth and softness. Feel all the knots unraveling from your belly, leaving it warm and relaxed.

Breathe down your back; breathe warmth into the muscles of your back. Feel all the tension and knots washing down and out its very base.

Breathe into your hips and legs. Feel tension washing down your legs and out through your feet and toes. Your legs feel warm and relaxed.

Your entire body, from your head all the way down to your toes, feels warm and relaxed. A wave of relaxation washes over you as you feel more and more relaxed.

It is time now for you to visit your Special Place in your mind.

Imagine that you are in a place where you feel safe and warm. Perhaps this is your room in your home.

...a Special Place for you – a safe place for you.

Imagine you are sitting on your bed at home. You feel warm and comfortable. Your bed is cozy and safe. You look around in your special place. Perhaps you see a stuffed animal or a favorite picture on the wall. You may have with you a blanket on your bed that you love. Notice what is here for you in your Special Place.

You feel safe here.

If you like, you can imagine that someone you love very much is here with you in your room. Take a moment now to experience this loving person here with you. Feel the love from your heart going into his or her heart and from his or her heart back into yours.

You are feeling safe and loved. This is a time for you to feel the love in your heart right now.

Breathe in softly and breathe out, feeling cozy in your safe place.

It is time now for you to leave your Special Place. You can visit this place any time you like in your imagination.

Begin to take some gentle breaths into your belly, feeling your muscles relaxing and warming. Breathe in softly in a wave of relaxation, and breathe out in a wave of relaxation. Breathe in softly and breathe out softly…

Take a moment now to appreciate yourself for taking this time to relax. Breathe in softly and breathe out softly…

If it is comfortable for you to do so, you may repeat to yourself, "I feel safe and loved. I feel safe and loved."

Breathe more deeply as you begin to wake up. Raise your arms above your head and shake your hands and fingers.

Take three breaths into your belly and open your eyes with a smile on your face.

Feel proud of yourself for doing this!

Heart Loving Rosebud

This is a time now for you to feel the loving power of your own beautiful heart.

Take a peaceful breath deep into your belly, and as you breathe out, let go of all tension.

Allow all the muscles of your body, from your head all the way down to your toes, to relax and become soft. Breathe in now in a wave of relaxation, and breathe out in a wave.

Bring your attention to your beautiful heart. If you like, you can place one or both of your hands on your heart, or just close your eyes and imagine how it feels. Perhaps you can feel some warmth coming from your heart. This is your very own loving heart energy. Your heart is so beautiful – just like a beautiful little flower.

Imagine in your heart is a soft and beautiful little rosebud. What color is this little rosebud? Breathe softly and imagine this rosebud opening up slowly and lovingly. Feel the love from deep in your heart spreading outwards through your body. The rosebud opens more and more fully until it is completely open and in full, magnificent bloom.

Feel this love as it spreads and washes through your entire mind, body, heart and spirit, creating a deep sense of love and peace within your whole self.

You have so much love in your heart and it needs to be shared!

Bring into your imagination the image of a person that you love very deeply. Imagine this person in detail. Imagine her face and eyes. Imagine a smile now on her face.

Begin to experience loving energy coming out from your beautiful heart and traveling into the heart of this special person. Perhaps this energy may have a color or be warm or glowing. What does it look like to you? What does it feel like?

Imagine this special person receiving your beautiful loving energy from your heart into her heart right now. You can see a smile on her face, and you know your heart energy is warming her heart right now. Perhaps you can imagine this person putting one or both of her hands over her heart.

With your next soft breath into your belly, you can imagine that beautiful loving energy is traveling back out from her heart and into your heart. See this heart energy entering your heart like a loving heart hug. You can feel the warmth and love deep in your heart from this special person.

Experience this now for a few moments...and while taking a gentle, soothing breath into your belly, you can bring a smile to your face!

Now, take a deep breath into your belly, and as you breathe out, you feel the power of your own loving heart. You feel peaceful now...and calm.

Begin to open your eyes. Stretch you arms above your head.

Garden River

This meditation will help guide you through the process of relaxing your mind and body.

Begin now by drawing your awareness to your breathing. Notice the rate and flow of your breath. Breathe in softly and deeply into your belly, and exhale out fully and completely.

Notice the coolness of the air as you breathe in through your nose and the warmth of the air as you breathe out through your nose.

Feel the comfort of your breath as you breathe deeply into your belly and exhale, letting go of tension.

Draw your awareness to the muscles of your body and begin to relax the top of your head. Allow the muscles of your face to let go and soften. Take a gentle breath in, and as you breathe out, release all tension from the muscles around your eyes, cheeks and jaw.

Allow your neck to let go of any holding and any tension. Feel how comfortable it is to let go of tension in your shoulders. Allow this tension to roll down your shoulders, down your arms and out through your fingertips.

Breathe softly now into your chest as your chest begins to open up, creating space and comfort.

Relax the muscles of your ribs and feel your ribs expanding in the front, sides and back of your body.

Breathe warmth into your belly as your belly rises softly and release all tension as you exhale.

Breathe into the muscles of your back, and as you breathe out, feel all of the tension wash down your spine and out its very base.

Breathe now into your pelvis and feel your pelvis relax and let go.

Become aware of your legs, and with your next deep exhalation, allow all the tension to wash down your legs and out through your toes.

Your body is feeling relaxed and comfortable.

Draw your attention now to your imagination. Allow your mind to be clear and empty.

Bring into your mind the image of yourself walking along a beautiful path with trees and flowers. The earth is soft and warm beneath your feet.

You walk peacefully along this path now, listening to the sounds in the environment, perhaps birds rustling in the leaves of trees.

You walk comfortably and peacefully along the path until you come to a garden gate. This is the most beautiful gate you have ever seen. The gate is covered with lovely flowers.

These are you favorite flowers. Take a moment now to admire and appreciate the beauty of flowers on the garden gate.

The sun is shining; it is a beautiful day. You can feel the warmth of the sun on your face and arms.

You open the gate now, step inside, and find yourself in the most beautiful garden you have ever visualized. This garden is here just for you.

Take some time to see what is in your garden. What treasures are here for you?

Begin to walk around your garden. Perhaps notice the flowers, a vegetable garden, or maybe beautiful trees and grass beneath your feet, as you walk peacefully and mindfully through your garden.

You walk over to the edge of a bank and notice a lovely river. Water is flowing gently along the river. You sit down under a big leafy tree, enjoying the shade. You rest comfortably on the bank by the river.

Breathe softly into your belly. As you exhale now, you are beginning to feel more calm.

Notice any worries that you might have in your mind.

You see beside you leaves that have fallen gracefully to the earth from the big tree. You pick up one of the leaves and place a worry in the leaf.

This leaf is just the right shape and size to hold your worry.

Gently leaning over the bank, you place this leaf in the river and watch it drift down the river...around the bend...and out of sight.

You pick up another leaf now and place another worry on this leaf. Leaning over the bank, you place this leaf in the river and watch it as it drifts down the river...around the bend...and out of sight.

One at a time you pick up leaves and place worries on the leaves, then place them gently and thoughtfully in the river, watching them all drift away...around the bend...and out of sight.

You can continue to do this until all your worries drift down the river...around the bend...and out of sight.

Little by little your mind begins to clear, creating space, calm, and a feeling of peace.

After all the worries have washed down the river, you take some time to simply sit and be by the river.

You look up at the sky and notice beautiful white fluffy clouds in the sky above. Perhaps you notice birds as they fly under the sun, the sun's rays glistening on their wings.

You are feeling peaceful and calm now.

It is time now for you to leave your garden. You stand up and begin to walk back.

Noticing the beauty around you, you come up to the garden gate, turn around, look at your garden, and feel again the warmth of the sun as you raise your arms upwards towards the sky.

Gather energy from the sun and feel this cleansing, healing energy wash through you.

You walk outside your garden gate now and close the gate behind you.

Turn again to gaze at the gate and the flowers that are here just for you.

You take a moment to appreciate this garden and know that you can return at any time.

You walk down the path now feeling refreshed and peaceful.

Draw your awareness back to your breathing. Notice the peaceful rhythm of your breath. Allow yourself to attend to your breathing.

Begin to take deeper cleansing breaths as you restore your energy, waking up mindfully from your meditation.

Take a moment now to appreciate yourself for taking this time to relax your body, mind, and heart.

Wake up feeling refreshed and rejuvenated.

Magic Garden

I invite you now to come on a journey into your imagination to visit a beautiful Magic Garden.

Take a couple breaths into your belly, and as you breathe out, let go of any tightness in your muscles. Shake your hands and wiggle your feet as you breathe in relaxation and breathe out tension.

Feel yourself becoming relaxed and peaceful.

Imagine you are walking along a beautiful path in the Magic Forest. You are on your way to the Magic Garden! There are pretty little flowers and small bushes on this special path.

You walk along, feeling relaxed and comfortable. The warm sun is shining on your face and arms. You swing your arms gently as you walk. Perhaps you can skip along your path, feeling the energy in your body.

You are feeling warm and very relaxed.

As you walk along the path, you see the Peace Tree! You can go up to her now if you like and give her a big hug. Feel her loving comfort now as you hug. Do you have any worries to give to the Peace Tree?

If you want, you can climb up to the branch that is holding the Worry Basket. Imagine yourself opening the basket and placing all of your worries inside. Now close the basket and leave it on the branch. The Peace Tree will take care of all your worries. Climb back down the tree and continue on your way to the Magic Garden.

Up ahead you see another tree. It is the Hugging Tree, and she is so happy that you have arrived. Open your arms wide and give her a big hug. Do you want to pat the little rabbit and climb around in the Hugging Tree? Imagine you are sitting in a cozy spot on the Hugging Tree and feeling her loving comfort.

You continue to walk along your path in the Magic Forest and come up to a garden gate. This is the gate to the Magic Garden. You have arrived! What does the gate look like? On this garden gate, you see pretty flowers that look happy. Perhaps they have smiling faces on them! What colors are your flowers?

Open the gate now and step inside the Magic Garden. This is the most beautiful garden you have ever seen. There are beautiful flowers and bushes. You see birds flying by overhead. The birds are singing happy songs. You feel peaceful.

Look at what is here in the Magic Garden. You begin to walk around your garden. Perhaps you skip...or dance.

You are feeling very free and happy here in your special garden.

As you walk along through the garden, you see a little place where you can plant your own little magic vegetable garden! Walk up to this special spot and sit down on your knees. Feel the warm earth with your hands. The warm sun is nourishing the soil.

Next to you is a little bucket of water, and next to that is a little bowl of magic seeds. These seeds are here just for you. Pick up one of the seeds. What does the seed feel like in your hand? Is it warm and soft, small or large? What kind of seed is this? Is it a fruit seed or vegetable seed...a chocolate seed? It can be anything you want.

Make a little hole in the soil. Plant the seed in your little garden and pat the soil lovingly with your hands. Now take some of the water from the pail and pour it over the seed. The sun is shining down on the seed in the soil, giving it nourishment and everything it needs to grow.

You look around in your vegetable garden and see things growing already. Perhaps there are tomatoes, cucumbers or carrots. Perhaps you see an apple tree...or...an ice cream tree! What is growing in your garden?

You feel peaceful and happy here.

You feel healthy and strong.

Lay back on the soft grass now and look up at the sky. Above you are some soft fluffy clouds. Notice the shapes of the clouds. Perhaps you see a bunny shape or the shape of a puppy. Just relax now, looking up at the clouds, and notice what you see.

You feel peaceful and happy.

You get up from the ground and begin to walk around your garden. The birds are over on a tree next to you, singing their songs and flapping their wings.

You feel very light and peaceful now.

Perhaps there is someone with you in your garden that you love. You take a moment to play with this person in the garden.

You feel very happy in your garden.

It is time now to leave your Magic Garden, so you wander over to the garden gate. You again look at the flowers on the garden gate and see their happy smiling faces. A warm feeling of joy and happiness washes over you.

You feel relaxed and happy.

Go outside your garden gate and close it behind you. Begin to walk back down the path in the Magic Forest and know that you can return to your Magic Garden in your imagination anytime you like.

Now it is time to wake up.

Take three deep breaths into your belly and stretch you arms above your head.

You feel wonderful!

Butterfly Garden

Let's begin by sitting in a comfortable spot in a cozy chair, or outside in a lovely spot in nature. Take a few deep breaths into your belly to help yourself feel more peaceful and quiet. Breathe the air in through your nose, feeling your belly expand, and exhale out all of the air through your nose or mouth.

Shake your arms and hands, and notice how each breath that you take helps you feel more and more relaxed.

If you like, you can stretch your arms up above your head and wiggle your elbows and hands. You can move your arms up and down as though you are flapping your very own butterfly wings. You can bring your hands to the top of your head and wiggle your fingers like little butterfly antennae.

Butterflies are wonderful and beautiful, just like you.

Imagine you are standing in front of the gate at the entrance to the Butterfly Garden. It is a sunny day and you can feel the warmth of the sun on your face. The gate is covered with beautiful, colorful flowers and lots and lots of butterflies. What colors are the flowers and butterflies?

These butterflies are waiting for you to open the gate so they may enter the Butterfly Garden with you. Open the gate now and step into the beautiful garden! Imagine that you are in the Butterfly Garden right now, where friendly beautiful butterflies are playing with new friends.

There are many colorful butterflies all around you, fluttering and flying in the bushes and flowers. Look! Here next to you is a yellow butterfly, sitting on a tiny purple flower. The flower looks very cozy to sit on. The petals of the flower are warm from the suns rays.

You look above your head and see other butterflies flying in the sky. They are having a really fun time, flapping their wings and wiggling their antennae. How many butterflies do you see?

Suddenly, a purple butterfly flies down to visit the yellow butterfly. The yellow butterfly is very shy, but he chooses to feel very courageous right now and wants to make a new friend. If you look closely, you can see both of these butterflies wiggling their antennae. This is how they talk to each other and invite each other to play.

The purple butterfly starts to fly back up to the sky with the yellow butterfly following him. Look at these two new friends now as they flutter and fly about with the other butterflies. Notice their happy faces and warm, lovely smiles.

You can imagine right now that you too are a beautiful butterfly! Imagine that you are sitting on a cozy warm purple flower and are hoping to make a new friend. What color are your butterfly wings? Can you feel your wings stretching and wiggling? How do you feel?

Oh, look above you! Here is the yellow butterfly fluttering down to say hello to you...and here is the purple butterfly too! Can you see the smiles on their faces? They are wiggling their antennae and inviting you to join them.

Imagine now that you flap your butterfly wings up and down and bring a beautiful smile to your face. Wiggle your antennae and start to fly up to the sky with your new butterfly friends. You feel courageous and happy.

Imagine that you are fluttering and flying around with all the butterflies in the sky. They are happy you are here! You are feeling free now and very happy that you made some new friends.

Imagine that you are flying and playing with your new butterfly friends for as long as you like. You have made new friends who will always be waiting to play with you in your Butterfly Garden.

It is time now for you to fly back to your cozy purple flower. Feel your butterfly wings flap as you flutter down and sit on the cozy purple flower.

Stretch your butterfly wings up above you and wiggle your antennae.

Bring a big smile to your face now. You can imagine your Butterfly Garden anytime you want to!

Take three breaths in and three breaths out. Feel proud of yourself!

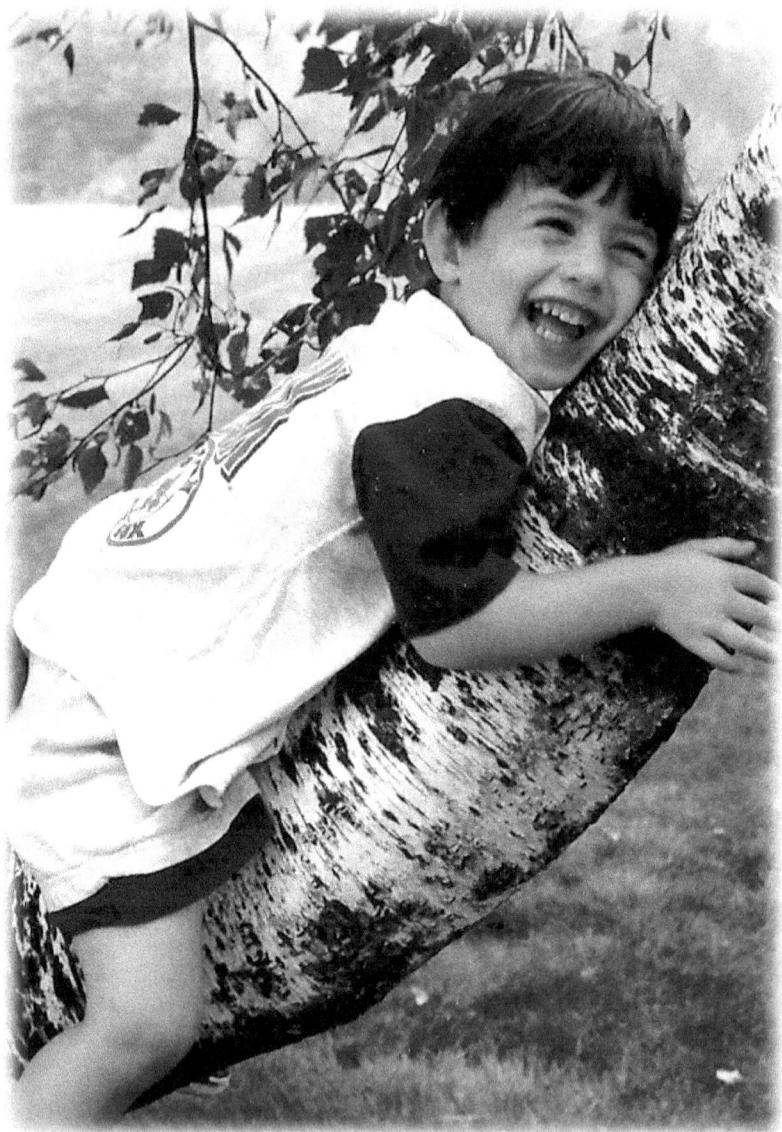

Magic Mountain

This is a time for you to feel strong and powerful!

Take a few deep breaths into your belly. As you breathe, you can relax all the muscles of your body, from your head all the way down to your feet and toes.

Shake your hands and shrug your shoulders. You feel comfortable and relaxed. Breathe in softly and breathe out softly. Each breath that you take helps you become more peaceful and calm.

Imagine yourself walking along a beautiful sunny path in the Magic Forest. You are on your way to the Magic Mountain! The sun is streaming through the trees, and everything in the forest is bright and beautiful. You see lots of flowers, bushes and trees. What colors are the flowers? Look! There is a family of birds sitting in a cozy nest in one of the bushes. You stop for a moment to smile at the birds. They are flapping their little wings in joy.

You continue to walk along the path and come to a special tree. It is the Peace Tree and she is here for you to give her all your worries. Give your special tree a big hug and feel her loving energy comfort you.

Climb up now and sit on one of the lowest branches. There is a Worry Basket there with your name on it waiting for you to place your worries inside. While up in the branch, you take all the worries that you might have now and place them in the basket. It is just the right size to hold all your worries. You close the top of the basket and let the Peace Tree hold it for you.

The Peace Tree will now take care of all these worries for you. You climb back down the tree and walk along the path.

Up ahead you see a beautiful mountain. This is the Magic Mountain! You stop and look up at the very top of the mountain. This mountain is powerful and strong, just like you.

Imagine walking up this mountain. Take a deep breath in...breathe out and relax. The sun is shining as you walk up your mountain. It is a beautiful day.

You see a little river next to you, and in the river are sweet birds washing and flapping their wings as they play. What colors are your birds? Do you hear singing or chirping from the birds? One little baby bird flies over and sits on your finger. You touch her head gently; her feathers feel so soft and cozy. She flies off and you continue to walk along the path and up your mountain. You can hear the sounds of the birds singing their songs.

As you walk along, you feel peaceful and strong.

Imagine that you are swinging your arms and breathing deeply. The air is clear and you feel so much energy and so strong!

You feel so free and happy!

You walk up the Magic Mountain and see more bushes and flowers. The flowers look like they have little smiles on their faces. They are happy and warm from the sun. You can feel the warm sun on your face and hands too. You bring a little smile to your face.

You feel free, happy and strong.

You walk up your path now and get to the very top of your Magic Mountain! Look! There is a comfortable place for you to sit on the earth. Maybe there is a glass of cold water and a snack. Little flowers and grass are here for you, just like a comfy, little bed. What colors are the flowers? You reach out and touch some of the petals with your fingers. Do they feel soft and warm? Is the grass cozy and soft?

You sit at the top of your Magic Mountain and look around you. You can see very far where there are mountains, valleys, and lots of birds flying around while singing.

You feel happy and peaceful. You feel very strong and powerful, just like the Magic Mountain!

You take some breaths in now, feeling strong and energetic. You breathe in, breathe out, and take some gentle breaths, feeling peaceful and calm.

It is time now for you to say, "Goodbye," to your Magic Mountain. You know that you can return and visit any time that you like.

Take three breaths into your belly and begin to wake up. You are feeling very strong and powerful.

Take a deep breath in now, and as you breathe out, say to yourself, "I am strong and powerful!"

Bring your arms above your head, breathe and stretch, repeating to yourself again, "I am strong and powerful!"

Take another deep breath in. Breathe out and feel good about yourself!

Magic Rainbow

Let's imagine sliding down the Magic Rainbow!

Imagine that you are sitting on soft, warm sand next to the sea at a beautiful beach. What color is the sand? The sea breeze is refreshing and ruffles your hair gently as it blows.

You are sitting right by the sea and notice next to you a little bird playing by the water's edge. What color is your bird? The breeze is ruffling the feathers of this little bird just like it ruffles your hair. You flap you arms around as if they are wings and begin to imitate the little bird in its play. The little bird chirps a few notes. You chirp these sounds back to the bird.

You are feeling happy here at the beach and feel like playing. You get up from the sand and splash around in the water with the little bird, happy that you have found a friend.

You look up above your head and notice a beautiful Magic Rainbow! This Magic Rainbow is bright, colorful, and as tall as a tree. At the bottom of the Magic Rainbow are little colorful stairs. You run over to these stairs and begin to climb up the rainbow. What color are your stairs? It is so easy to go up the Magic Rainbow, and you run up the stairs to the very top.

The little bird flies over to you, chirps a few notes, and then begins to slide down the other side of the Magic Rainbow. You are feeling happy and free up here on the Magic Rainbow.

The breeze ruffles up your hair. Now it is your turn to play "sliding down the bow." You sit down on the Magic Rainbow and it hugs you safely as you slide down the bow. You can slide fast or slow, however you like; you are in complete control as you slide down the rainbow into the soft beach sand at the bottom.

The little bird is waiting for you at the bottom of the Magic Rainbow. This is fun! Together, you and your new friend, the little bird, race back to the colorful stairs on the other side of your Magic Rainbow and play on it for as long as you like. You feel happy and free.

It is time now for you to leave your rainbow. Say, "Goodbye," to your friend, the little bird...and to the Magic Rainbow. Anytime you want to feel happy and free, you can go to your imagination and play "sliding down the bow" on your Magic Rainbow.

Take three breaths into your belly now and raise your arms above your head. Wiggle your fingers and bring a smile to your face. Good for you!

Magic Star Ride

I invite you to come on a wonderful journey in the Magic Forest to search for treasure.

Take a relaxing breath into your belly. If you like, you can place your hands on your belly and feel it rise when you breathe in and get smaller when you breathe out, just like a balloon. You can make a soft sound like, "Ahhhh," with your breath as you breathe out. Try that with your next breath out; breathe in, and as you breathe out, say, "Ahhhh."

Now, scrunch up your face and eyes for a moment, open your mouth as big as you can and wiggle your tongue. If you like, you can shake your hands and feet gently as though you are shaking all the tension out of your body.

You are feeling free and light.

Imagine now that you are walking along a special path in the Magic Forest. You are very happy to be in the Magic Forest because you are going to search for treasure! There is a special treasure box with something magical inside, hiding in the Magic Forest just for you. You are on your way right now to discover it.

You walk along the path, swinging your arms above your head. You are barefoot and feel the sun warming the soft earth beneath your toes as you walk along. If you like, you can skip, jump or dance along your path. Take a deep breath into your belly and breathe out softly.

You are feeling free and light.

You look around you and notice pretty flowers, trees and bushes all along the path. There is a special green bush with little berries on it right in front of you on the path. On one of the branches is a bird having a tasty snack of berries. What color is your bird? The bird whistles a happy song when she sees you and flaps her wings. Can you imagine you are flapping your wings just like the little bird?

You look closely at your bird and notice something bright and shiny that she is carrying under her wings. What treasure could this be? It looks like a bright star! Your new bird friend flies off down the path and you follow her, skipping along the path, feeling free and light. She is going to take you to the treasure box.

As you walk along your path, you see a beautiful tree next to a little river. It is the Peace Tree and she is here for you to give her all your worries. Give the Peace Tree a big hug and feel her loving energy comfort you.

The bird flies up to the lowest branch, sits down, and begins to whistle for you to come. Climb up now and sit on the lowest branch. There is a small basket with your name on it. This is the Worry Basket and it is here for you to fill with all your worries.

Imagine yourself placing all your worries into this basket right now. If you like, you can say what each worry is and then imagine placing it in the basket for the Peace Tree to take care of. Take a moment to do this now. The Peace Tree will take care of all these worries for you.

You climb safely back down the tree and thank your Peace Tree for being here for you.

You are feeling free and light. All your worries are gone and you feel happy.

You skip down your path and see your bird flying in front of you. It looks like the shiny star treasure that it has under its wings is sparkling now. What colors are the sparkles? The shiny treasure is carrying the bird. It looks fun!

You walk along your path, maybe skipping or dancing. Take a deep breath into your belly, breathe out and feel all your muscles relax – just like pudding.

Look! Your bird is sitting on a beautiful, colorful box right in the middle of the path. It is the treasure box that is waiting here just for you!

Your bird hops off of the box and onto your shoulders, and you bend down to take a closer look at the treasure box. You see jewels all over it. What do the jewels look like? What colors are they? Do they glimmer and sparkle? Do they shine or glow? What is your treasure box made of?

You are feeling very happy now, and you open the top of the box to look inside. Look! There, inside, is a shiny Magic Star just for you! It sparkles and shines brightly, and you take it out of the treasure box. What color is your star? Is it warm or cold in your hands?

You see that the Magic Star is big enough to hold you, and you climb onto it, feeling safe and cuddled. Imagine now that your Magic Star carries you up and gracefully glides through the air.

You are having so much fun floating through the air on your star. Your Magic Star dances around the Magic Forest, and you feel free and light. You can see your bird on her own star dancing along next to you in the air.

Take a few moments to imagine yourself floating freely through the air on your Magic Star.

You are feel safe and happy.

You feel free and light.

The Magic Star glides gently back to the earth, and you get off and sit down next to the treasure box. The box is sparkling. You take your Magic Star and place it back into the box for now. You close the top of the box, feeling free and light.

You get up and begin to swing your arms and skip and dance back down your path. You pass the Peace Tree and leave all your worries on the branches of the tree because you do not need these worries anymore!

You feel free and light.

You see the green bush on the path now, and your bird is sitting on one of the branches having a snack of a berry. You say, "Goodbye," to your bird, and your bird whistles a happy song.

It is time to leave your Magic Forest for now. You can return in your imagination anytime you like to visit your Magic Forest and have a ride on your Magic Star.

Begin to take a deep breath into your belly. All the muscles of your body are feeling soft and relaxed. Take another deep breath in, filling yourself with healthy air and energy.

You feel free, light and wonderful.

Take three breaths into your belly and wake up.

Stretch your arms above your head now, and wiggle your fingers and toes.

Bring a big smile to your face and feel good about yourself!

Be a Bird

Let's Imagine!

We are now going to imagine being a bird!

Sit down in a comfortable place, perhaps in a cozy chair or a beautiful spot in nature. Take a soft breath into your belly and notice how you are able to begin to relax. Raise your arms up above your head and bring them back down like you are flapping your wings.

Begin now to imagine that you are walking in a Magic Garden. It is a beautiful sunny day, and you can feel the warmth of the sun on your face and arms as you walk. You feel completely safe here in the Magic Garden.

You begin to hear lovely birdsongs that are sweet music to your ears. You stop by a pretty green bush with small branches and flowers on it. What colors are the flowers? Take a moment to appreciate their beauty and smiling faces!

As you look more closely inside the bush, you see a small bird nest nestled into the center. Look! There are baby birds wiggling around and chirping for their breakfast. There is a mother bird feeding her sweet baby birds some tasty berries. She is chattering and calming them with her birdsong.

The baby birds are getting ready for their very first flight, and you are here to watch! Notice how the mother bird lovingly urges her babies to the edge of the nest as the baby birds begin to flap their wings and wiggle their tails. There is a gentle breeze in the air, and immediately the little courageous birds take flight out of the nest, flying around and above you.

Take a deep breath into your belly and begin to feel what it is like to be a bird. You can feel their courage! The little baby birds return to their warm nest, snug, cozy and safe.

Imagine yourself right now as a baby bird nestled inside this cozy nest! What color bird are you? Feel the gentle breeze ruffling in your soft feathers and under your imaginary bird wings. You feel a gentle loving nudge against your back and hop to the edge of your nest.

You are feeling strong and powerful today and are ready to fly. Feel the excitement in your heart as your courage grows stronger! In your imagination, you begin to flap your bird wings and feel the rush of powerful energy wash through you. This is your moment to fly! Flap your wings and lift off from the nest, knowing you have everything you need to succeed.

The gentle breeze lifts you up above the bush. As you flap your wings, you feel completely safe and free.

Imagine yourself gliding along through the air now, dipping, twirling and flapping, experiencing a wonderful feeling of being free.

You are a beautiful bird. What colors are you? Are you big or small? Are your wings long or wide?

Spend some time in your imagination flapping your wings and feeling what it is like to have fun flying!

It is time now for you to go back to the nest. You glide back through the air to the edge of the cozy warm nest. You hop back into the bird nest now, feeling your courage and strength.

You can return anytime you like in your imagination to your Magic Garden and visit the cozy warm nest of the baby birds.

Take a soft breath into your belly as you wake up from your bird imagery. Notice how you are able to create a wonderful feeling of being free just by using your imagination.

Raise your arms above your head and flap your wings! Take a deep breath into your belly and bring a smile to your beautiful face.

Feel proud of yourself!

Energy Ball

Let's relax together.

Wiggle your arms and fingers, and wiggle your feet and toes. Scrunch up your face and wiggle your tongue. Take a deep breath into your belly, and as you breathe out, bring a smile to your face. Feel the smile as it flows through your whole body.

You are feeling more relaxed.

Imagine right above your head is your very own Energy Ball! This Energy Ball is full of healing energy just for you. What does this healing energy look like? Do you see tiny hearts, happy suns, or shiny stars? Is it a glowing light or a soft cloud? It can be anything YOU want!

Bring your hands above your head to touch your Energy Ball (or, you can imagine doing this in your mind). Can you feel the energy in your fingers? What does the energy feel like? Do your hands feel tingly or warm? The energy feels good!

Now, imagine tiny hearts, happy suns, shiny stars, glowing light, or a soft cloud flowing down from your Energy Ball, into your head, and all the way down to your toes. This feels wonderful! They are here to soothe all your aches and pains.

Now, think of a certain place inside you that needs healing and comfort. Maybe you have sniffles or your tummy aches. Or maybe you have a cut on your finger or a blister on your foot. Feel this healing energy flowing through you and into this place right now. This energy knows just where to go!

Are the tiny hearts giving the ache hugs? Are the happy suns warming the ache away? Are the shiny stars bringing cooling relief to the pain? Is the glowing light showing the aches how to fly away? Is the soft cloud wrapping around the ache and carrying the ache away? What do you see?

Imagine this place being healed. You feel better!

Take three soft breaths into your belly. It is time now to wake up. You can imagine your Energy Ball anytime you like and bring healing energy to any place in your body at any time. You have the power to help yourself feel better!

Good for you!

Energy Shield

This is a time now for you to feel your own personal protective power. You have the ability to call upon your inner strength in your mind, body and heart whenever you need it.

This Energy Shield is a powerful imagery. When you imagine an Energy Shield around you, you create the ability to let in good energy and to keep out what doesn't feel good.

In this imagery, you will choose what you allow to come in through your Energy Shield. This Energy Shield is protection to place around yourself whenever you feel the need.

Begin now to draw your awareness to your breath. Allow your breath to be a relaxing energy in your body. Feel each breath as it washes through you, filling your body with precious oxygen and strengthening your mind, body and heart.

Breathe deep into your belly and feel this breath wash into your head and face. Feel this breath as it soothes all the muscles deep within and around your eyes. Perhaps you can feel all the muscles of your face becoming soft and relaxed.

Breathe deep into your neck and shoulders, and down into your arms, hands and fingers. Breathe all the tension out from your muscles and notice how your body is becoming more relaxed.

Breathe down your back and feel all the tension wash down and out the very base of your spine.

Breathe into your chest and heart space, and feel an abundance of space in your chest as you breathe. Take a moment to experience the healthy beating of your own loving heart.

Breathe into your belly and feel your belly becoming soft and warm. Breathe into your hips and feel all tension washing out of your body as you exhale. Breathe down your legs now and feel this breath as it washes into your feet and toes.

Breathe now from your head all the way down to your toes. Take a moment to enjoy this feeling of deep relaxation and peace. With each breath that you take, you become more and more powerful.

Begin now to imagine that all around you is a powerful Energy Shield. You are completely safe. This Energy Shield is here for your protection and safety.

What does this Energy Shield look like? What size is it so that it can fully protect you? Does it have a color? Is the energy glowing or sparkling?

Imagine your very own Energy Shield in any way that you like!

Nothing can enter into this Energy Shield without your permission. Begin to notice that whatever is outside of it stays outside. You have the power to allow into the shield only what feels right or good to you. Take some time now to experience being protected by your Energy Shield.

What do you want to allow to come in? As you allow something in, notice how it makes you feel. You can breathe out anything that does not feel right to you. Take a breath and breathe it right out of the Energy Shield, right now. You have complete control over what you let in.

Take some soothing breaths now and simply be inside your Energy Shield, feeling safe and protected. Breathe from your head all the way down to your toes and feel the strength of your own mind, body and heart. Experience this for as long as you like.

Begin to take a few deep breaths as you wake up from your Energy Shield imagery. You are feeling powerful and safe. You have the ability to create your Energy Shield any time you need it.

Stretch your arms above your head and shake your hands and feet.

You are strong and powerful!

One Minute Journeys

Magic Fluffy Clouds

Visualize where an ache is hiding in your body. Did you find it? Where is it?

Now imagine that a magic fluffy cloud is wrapped around the ache. The ache is inside the fluffy cloud.

You can make the fluffy cloud as big as you need to hold the ache. The fluffy cloud is here to help you.

What color is your fluffy cloud? See it in your mind.

This fluffy cloud is ready to carry the ache away.

Now imagine this fluffy cloud becoming softer, fluffier, lighter and flying away! It is carrying the ache away with it. See the color becoming lighter and lighter until it is white. Visualize this until the fluffy cloud is tiny and out of sight.

Take a full breath throughout your mind, body and heart. You feel better!

Ball of Soothing Ice Water/Snow

Imagine above your head is a big ball of soothing ice. What color is the ice? Is it blue or white?

Imagine soothing ice water washing down over you, from your head all the way to your toes. It feels cool and soothing. It is so refreshing.

Imagine the ice water washing into all your aches and pains, cooling and soothing them away.

Rosebud

Take a peaceful breath deep into your belly, and as you breathe out, let go of all tension.

Now imagine in your heart is a soft and beautiful little rosebud. What is the color of this little rosebud?

With each breath that you take, imagine this rosebud beginning to open up slowly and lovingly.

Begin to feel love from deep in your heart spreading outwards through your body as the rosebud opens more and more fully until the rose is completely open and in full magnificent bloom.

Feel this love as it spreads and washes through your entire mind, body, heart and spirit, creating a deep sense of love and peace within your whole self.

Take your hands, place them over your heart, and bring a smile to your face.

Heart Hug

Take one or both of your hands and place them softly over your heart on your chest. Close you eyes and breathe softly into your belly.

You can feel the warmth from your heart energy under your hands and fingers. This loving energy is always there in your heart, ready to give you a loving heart hug.

Bring a smile to your face. You feel loved.

Glowing Ball of Magical Light

Imagine above your head is a glowing ball of magical light. Perhaps it is golden, purple, or white.

Imagine now that this light is washing down like a waterfall into your head, neck and shoulders; down into your arms, hands and fingers; down your back; down into your chest, heart space and belly; and down into your hips, legs, feet and toes.

Your whole body, from your head all the way down to your toes, is filled with this magical light.

This light is waking up the powerful healing cells in your body.

Now imagine this magical light washing back up through your toes; up through your feet, legs and hips; up through your back; up through your belly and into your chest and heart space; up through your fingers, hands and arms; and up through your shoulders, neck and head. It is washing up like a waterfall back into the glowing ball of magical light above your head.

You feel wonderful!

Special Place

Imagine a Special Place where you feel safe and secure.

This might be your room at home, a beautiful garden, a favorite beach, or a make-believe place.

Imagine whatever YOU want.

What is here in your Special Place? Is there a favorite pet or someone who loves you?

You can invite anyone you want into your Special Place.

You are completely safe and loved here.

You feel cozy and protected.

You feel safe and secure.

Imagine being in your Special Place right now.

Energy Shields

Imagine above you is a glowing light. Now imagine special light energy flowing down from the light and surrounding you in a protective Energy Shield. What is your energy made of? What color is your Energy Shield? How does it feel to be inside of it? You are completely safe inside this Energy Shield.

~

Imagine you have an Energy Shield power button in your hand. When you press the button, a magical Energy Shield appears all around you to protect you! Squeeze your hand now and activate the shield! You are safe and secure inside your Energy Shield right now. Just squeeze your hand to de-activate it. You can turn this on or off whenever you want!

~

Imagine that you have in your hand a magical Energy Shield. It has a little handle on it for you to hold. This Energy Shield is very light and easy for you to move around. What does it look like? Maybe it is covered with glowing lights, sparkling jewels or white stars. Raise the shield above your head so it protects you like an umbrella. A stream of protective energy flows all around you. Now place the Energy Shield on the earth and go sit inside it. Imagine your shield flying up into the air and carrying you away from all fears. You are completely safe inside this Energy Shield right now.

Story of Danielle

Share the remarkable story of a child as she taps into her mind, body, heart and soul to create unity and power within for self-healing.

This story is about Danielle, an Israeli child of age fifteen who underwent glaucoma surgery in February of 2012 at Ichilov Medical Center in Tel Aviv. She has been suffering from this condition since she was a small child and has experienced multiple surgeries, check-ups, medical procedures, and a tremendous amount of stress. I recommended she use my Children's Guided Imagery CD before, during, and after surgery in order to do the following: assist her in reducing pain and anxiety, create a safe place to go to when she feels fear, and promote recovery.

Danielle listened to my Children's Guided Imagery CD for several nights prior to her hospital stay. She chose to listen before falling asleep and primarily focused on her two favorite guided imageries, *Special Place* and *Heart Loving*. Each night, she fell asleep more quickly and easily, conveying feelings of relaxation and peace. She described how the peacefulness stayed with her all day. As a result, she did not need to listen to the CD in mornings at all.

Danielle's mom: "She felt more confident about herself in general, and specifically toward her ability to help the condition of her eye."

She felt peaceful and relaxed during a blood draw, completely the opposite response of past experiences. I visited her in the hospital the night before the surgery and observed a calm, happy, and mentally positive child. My CD helped her feel empowered during her hospital experience.

Danielle: "The meditation I liked and felt most bonded with was *Special Place*. When I listened to this meditation, I got a sense of security and love. When I was in the hospital, I succeeded in imagining myself at home in my room where I felt confident and secure. I also was able to relax my body so my soul felt calm and peaceful towards the surgery. In the meditation *Heart Loving*, I felt power being transferred to me, and I felt stronger without fear towards the surgery."

Two weeks after the surgery, Danielle was still using my CD at bedtime, especially if she felt anxious, because it helped her achieve peace and fall asleep quickly. This was a very successful integration of imagery into daily life! Danielle took advantage of her innate capacity for self-healing by tapping into her mind, body, heart and soul to create unity and power within.

Fast-forward four weeks: Danielle was preparing for a post-surgery procedure to correct the lens. Spontaneously, she began utilizing my Children's Guided Imagery CD to prepare for the surgery and re-create a sense of peace and control. Danielle's mom related that this CD opened up a new world to Danielle. She continues not only to experience less fear and anxiety, but also to learn about herself on a very deep level.

Danielle's mom: "The importance of this whole process is that Danielle has become more aware of herself and what she needs in order to help her body heal."

Fast forward to the present: Danielle continues to integrate my Children's Guided Imagery CD into her life with confidence. She now reads and loves the guided imagery scripts from "Magic Forest Hugging Tree." In addition, Danielle's mom created a beautiful image of light and healing in her own mind to share with Danielle. The results? Miraculous!

Danielle: "My mom closes her eyes while I'm closing mine, thinking of light, of healing, and surprisingly, it decreases my eye pressure."

Good for you Danielle!

Testimonials

"Ava was having a difficult time going to sleep at night, so Laura personalized a children's CD of guided meditations to help her relax while going to bed. Listening to Laura's calming voice and imagery became a part of Ava's nightly routine. She even had her own favorite meditations she looked forward to hearing at bedtime. Plus, I was able to enjoy the guided imagery as I put her to bed, which provided both a special bonding activity with my daughter and a nice way for me to wind down in the evening as well!"

Lisa, mother of three-year-old Ava - USA

~

"I love your CDs and the kids know you well, even if they have not spent time with you. When I brought it out for Eliza to listen, she got all excited! She listened to it with her earphones and stayed put until it was over. Such concentration this one; I asked her how she felt and she said... 'Everything is quiet; I like playing with the pink ball and thinking about butterflies. It makes me feel peaceful.'"

Kristin, mother of six-year-old Eliza - USA

~

"Danielle felt more confident about herself in general, and specifically toward her ability to help her eye's condition."

Nili, mother of fifteen-year-old Danielle – Israel

"The meditation that I felt the most bonding and liking for was *Special Place*. When I listened to this meditation I got a sense of security and love. When I was in the hospital, I succeeded to imagine that I am home in my room where I feel confident and secure. I also succeeded to relax my body so my soul felt relaxed and peaceful towards the surgery. In the meditation *Heart Loving*, I felt the power that was transferred through me and I felt stronger with no fear towards the surgery. In addition, my mom closed her eyes while I closed mine, thinking of light and healing, and surprisingly it decreased my eye pressure."

Danielle, fifteen years old – Israel

About the Author

Laura Hoffman, B.S., is a guided imagery expert and mind/body medicine skills specialist with over 36 years of experience training and counseling children and adults. She has advanced course training from the Mind/Body Medical Institute of Harvard Medical School and a massage therapy degree.

A pioneer in the use of guided imagery and meditation with children, Laura began teaching courses in high schools and preschools in 1975. She continues to bring this practice and its associated healing benefits into her whole life, witnessing remarkable results as she shares expertise with her own children and clients.

Throughout her career, Laura has created hundreds of guided imagery scripts and recordings. Further, she has designed guided imagery CD/script training programs for medical centers. Her work is enthusiastically received around the world.